MW00874723

45 Lazy Eye Exercises

Eye Patch Exercises To Improve
Vision for Those Who Suffer
from Amblyopia

Tammie Taylor

Published by TaylordFit
Memphis, TN 38134
Copyright © 2009 by Tammie Taylor

45 Lazy Eye Exercises
Eye Patch Exercises to Improve Vision for Those Who Suffer
from Amblyopia

ISBN: 144865601X
EAN-13: 9781448656011

This book is dedicated to my daughter, Jessica Ruth, whose courage is an inspiration to all. You mean the world to me. May God forever bless you.

~ INTRODUCTION ~

In November 2006, I learned that my six year old daughter suffered from a condition called amblyopia. Prior to this time, I had no idea what amblyopia was. What I thought would be an in and out visit at the optometrist's office turned out to be more than that.

Prior to this discovery, my husband and I had been alerted by my daughter's school that she had failed an eye pre-screening test. Therefore, we went ahead and scheduled a visit at the local optometrist's office. We made an eye appointment with the intent that she would just need a pair of glasses due to possible near-sightedness, which ran in our families. However, we were shocked and saddened to hear that she suffered from amblyopia.

Amblyopia, which is also known as "lazy eye", is a condition in which one has a reduction in vision in one eye for an unknown reason. The eye is perfectly healthy, but for some reason, the vision in that eye is not clear and thus the brain has partially cut off its use of it.

In order to begin restoring vision to the eye, one has to re-train their brain to begin using that particular eye in conjunction with the other eye. Due to the fact that the eye is being used less, the muscles in that particular eye are weak and need to also be strengthened.

The whole process to regain vision in the affected eye does not happen overnight and can be a lengthy process. The most common treatment that is used today for amblyopia is eye patch therapy.

Eye patching involves using an ophthalmic patch to cover the non-affected eye so that no light can penetrate through it. This allows vision from the eye that is not patched to be utilized. This will cause the affected eye to be the primary eye that is used while the patch is worn.

The length that a patch should be worn depends on the severity of the condition and any recommendations given by your particular doctor. My daughter wears her patch for nearly two hours a day. Others may wear their patch for a much longer timeframe. Consultation from a primary doctor on treatment frequency and duration is recommended.

When my doctor first introduced us to the idea of wearing the eye patch, it took a lot of acceptance from all of us. Most children hate the idea of a patch, especially if they have to wear it in a public setting. Thankfully so, we could limit our patching to wearing it only at home, although we still do run into problems getting our daughter to wear the patch on a consistent basis. I am sure that there are parents who have small toddlers or babies who are also required to wear eye patches daily. Because a child this young cannot understand the significance of the patch, it is very likely that they may try to pull it off of their eye throughout the entire day. No matter how old your child is, you will likely run into issues with them not wanting to patch.

However, what made eye patching more bearable for us was finding exercises that could be done while wearing the patch that were both fun and enjoyable.

When we first searched for exercises to do, it was pretty difficult. We just wanted ideas of activities that we could do with our child to make patching time more effective. We were advised to do near-sighted activities by our doctor's office. However, we wanted suggestions from other people who had experienced the same thing that we were now experiencing. There was very little information available. Even our optometrist's office lacked those types of resources. After trying out so many different activities with my daughter, I wanted to compile as much information as possible to help others who were facing this same type problem.

In this book, you will find a collection of 45 eye patching activities that you can do from home as a part of your patch therapy sessions. This is written from a parent's perspective and is intended to serve as a place for ideas on activities that you can consider doing while patching to assist in improving your child's vision.

The intended audiences for this book are parents, interested parties, and/ or those that suffer from amblyopia. However, the ideas covered in this book can be tailored to your own needs.

Please note that we are not medical physicians and are only providing information gathered from our own personal experience. As always, you should consult with your physician regarding your own personal medical condition.

Before we get started with the list of near-sighted activities, here is a collection of tips or suggestions that you may want to apply during any patch sessions with your child to ensure they are more effective.

EYE

PATCHING

TIPS

CONSISTENCY

It is important that you begin to setup a daily routine of patching with your child. If your doctor has suggested that you patch for a certain length of time, then it is important for you to stick to it as much as possible.

It can be difficult to get your child to put the patch on, however, if this is done on a consistent basis, then they will be more willing to wear the patch.

Setting aside the time and getting your child focused on performing these activities can be difficult especially if your child has other daily activities that are also important, like school, sports, or homework. However, the more consistent you are, the greater your results will be and the happier you will be with the progress that you make.

ENVIRONMENT

Tip 2

Be sure to perform any activities around a quiet, well lit area to get maximum results. This will allow you to reduce any extra strain to the eye.

If your child is performing activities while sitting, ensure that they are using good posture. If they are sitting slouched over, this will cause additional strain to their neck, which will cause them to be frustrated during the patching session.

If your child has trouble concentrating, then try to limit things that would distract them, like television or radio. You can consider playing soft calming music in the background while they are patching. Another idea is to perform your patch activities outside on a nice, breezy day. This will give your child an opportunity to experience a more relaxed environment while patching.

POSITIVE COMPLIMENTS

Tip 3

As your child is progressing and working through various exercises, be sure to provide positive reinforcement. It will help them have a more positive attitude towards wearing a patch.

Give them a compliment even for the smallest thing and reassure them that you are there to help them with any activity that they need some assistance with. Nurture them with extra love and kisses during this time.

If they "mentally" believe that they can do something, then nothing will be able to stop them from doing it. Instill as much confidence and encouragement in your child while they are patching. This will help to give a more positive attitude about patching and about life in general.

KEEP A JOURNAL

Tip 4

Keep a small journal while patching to record the activities that you do and to document any issues that you notice so that you can discuss them with your doctor. The journal will allow you to notice levels of progress as you go day by day. This will help you to notice how your child is progressing even without you having to ask your doctor. If your child was not able to do something last week, but now they are, then you will then be able to notice the change.

This simple idea will keep you and your child motivated along the way. It will also help to document areas of concern that you can discuss with your doctor later. Usually, we only get a small amount of time to discuss issues with our doctor. Therefore, we want to make it count by being able to ask questions based upon the information that you have documented. It is so much easier to recall information if it is written down than from memory.

TAKE YOUR TIME

Tip 5

Never rush through an activity. Try to take your time. Remember that you should tailor any activity to meet your child's condition. You do not have to follow the rules exactly. If it takes your child longer than average to do a specific task, then it's okay to slow down to their own pace.

If your child is engaged with an activity and does not wish to continue, then you can always choose another. Children often get restless and may tend to whine or complain if they are unhappy. The way to combat that is to introduce a new activity that they enjoy or that will spark their interest.

Also, try to remember to patch when your child is alert and is not sleepy or hungry. If they are sleepy and tired, then they will probably be frustrated and unwilling to patch. This will definitely help to ensure that you can complete your patching session more effectively.

TRY THE ACTIVITES YOURSELF

Tip 6

One of the easiest things that you can do with your child is to wear a patch and perform the activities together. This will help your child feel more comfortable and allow you to see things from their viewpoint. This will also strengthen your parental bond even greater.

Patching with your child allows you to spend more quality time with your kids. During this time, you get the benefit of working on activities together and having fun doing simple things. Your family bond will be greater as you will be gaining what most American families lack in these times, which are healthy family relationships.

Another thing that you can do to build even more relationships is to participate in patching groups so you child can play with other kids who also patch. If you can find someone in your area to start a group with, then this can be great for your child to connect with other kids.

CREATE A REWARD SYSTEM

Tip 7

Create a progress chart for your child and provide a reward if they accomplish a specific goal or task. An example of this is to create a chart where you put stickers on it for every day that your child patches. Another example could be a sticker is put on the chart every time your child completes a certain activity while patching. After a number of days have passed, then you can take them out for ice cream or their favorite treat as a reward.

The back of this book has an example of an activity chart that you can use to record what your child is doing. Your chart can be similar to this. However, you may want to make it so that it is large enough for your child to understand how they are progressing as well.

Allow your child to create it with you and put stickers on it once they complete an activity.

DECORATE THE PATCH

Give your child the opportunity to select their own patch and decorate it. You can either choose to order a patch that has a pre-made theme, like a frog or lady bug. There are some websites on the Internet, where you can buy a certain patch theme. Just think of your child's favorite animal and surprise them with it at your next patching session.

Another option is to decorate an ordinary patch on your own. This will help your child feel more comfortable when patching since they will actually like what they are wearing. You can either choose the black pirate patch to decorate or one of the stick on patches, the choice is yours.

These are tips to help make patching time much easier for your child. Try your best to follow these guidelines with your child as you see fit. It will help your child to accept patching better and be more motivated to perform any activities during patching. Now, that we have discussed some tips on eye patching; let's now move into the eye patching exercises.

The exercises that are presented over the next several pages are activities to help spark ideas on different things that you can do with your child. These are exercises that we have done with our child since she began patching. You can pick one or all of the exercises included and create a daily schedule of exercises to be performed.

These activities are also designed to give you a source of information so that you can plan out your child's therapy session. As always, change up any activity that you need to in accordance with your child's capability. Just make the session fun and interesting and that will give you greater results.

PATCH ACTIVITIES

CIRCLE THE LETTER

This activity works well for children who are old enough to recognize letters and numbers. To do this activity, gather a sheet of paper that contains typed written text. You can tear out a magazine article and use that if you desire.

Now, ask your child to circle every time they see the letter "a" in the text. However, the key is that they have to keep the pencil on the paper. They would underline the entire text and each time they see the specific letter, they would loop around it.

If your child cannot see the letters, print off a sheet of text from your computer with as large of a font that is needed for them to be able to see the letters. We started off with fonts as large as 16 point and gradually lowered the font size as vision improved.

COLOR THE O's

This activity is a variation of the previous activity. You will still need to have a sheet of paper with typed words. The difference is that you will need for your child to fill in every letter "O" or whatever you choose with any color that they desire.

They can use a pen, crayon, or marker for this activity. Just allow your child to be creative by selecting the colors that they wish to use.

FOLLOW THE PEN

To perform this activity, hold a pen or pencil in the air. Then, have your child focus his or her eyes on the ballpoint portion of the pen. Move the pen very slowly. While moving the pen, ensure that your child's eyes follow it. Make sure that your child does not move their head as they are following the pen.

Stop movement and see how quickly your child's eyes stop movement. As you get more advanced, make alphabet letters in the air with your pen and see if your child can guess the letter that you made.

EYE CHART

This activity involves using a small eye chart that contains uppercase alphabet letters that are spaced apart from each other. This is not something that you have to obtain from your doctor. You can easily create one from any word processing program or download an example off of the Internet.

You will just need to hang it on a wall and have your child focus on the chart while steadily walking backwards and forward until they can no longer see the chart.

Once they reach this threshold, have your child read off the letters that they see. As you get more advanced, then you can have your child skip certain lines to read or skip every other letter to read off the chart. An even more advanced technique would be to have your child read the letters while they are distracted with another activity. An example of this is to having your child hop up and down while reading the eye chart.

READING

Reading can also serve as a great means to improve vision while patching. All you need to do is to grab a copy of a favorite book that your child can read from.

If your child cannot read small print, then grab a large print book from your local library to use. Most libraries have a large print section for visually impaired members. Your only challenge would be to find interesting children's stories that are available in large print.

If your child is not old enough yet to read, then you can use picture books as an alternative to reading books. When using picture books, ask your child to point to objects on a page or to count the number of certain set of objects that he/ she sees on a specified page.

THE TRADITIONAL MATCH OR MEMORY GAME

The standard card game of matching is also a great activity that you can play with your child during patch time. You can use the deck of cards just like in the traditional game of match. Spread out the cards on a table and take turns trying to find a mate. "Memory" cards can also be used as an alternative.

Just take turns finding the mates for the cards. You may have to assist as needed to help your child with mates if they have a problem seeing the cards or if they have issues with visual memorization. However, this game gives really good practice with developing visual memorization skills.

LACING CARDS

Lacing or sewing cards are little cards that one can use to practice learning to sew or knit. They are available in different shapes and contain holes around the outer edge. These cards can be purchased from just about any retailer that has a craft department. The goal is to have your child loop a single string through the holes on the cards.

Have your child try each of the different stitches available (standard or cross stitch). Once completed, have your child unravel the stitches.

It may take a minute for your child to get the hang of it, but once they get used to it, I am sure that it will be one of their favorite activities. You can also have a race with your child to see who can lace the cards first and unravel them for extra fun.

BEADING

Who doesn't like to bead or make jewelry? It's definitely a fun activity that your child will enjoy. Obtain some beads and string from your local craft store. Try to look for beads and string that is not too tiny for your child as they may have trouble stringing beads if they too small. Have your child loop the beads through the string to make his or her own bracelet or necklace.

If you are using a table or countertop to bead, then make sure that the pattern on the table is not too busy. You will need enough contrast to ensure that your child can see the beads.

PLAY BALL

Playing sports can be a great activity to support eye patching. However, you do not have to participate in any sport that may be too complicated for eye patching, like football. As long as you have a ball that you can play with, then that is really all you need.

Rolling or playing catch with a ball is a great way to not only have fun, but help to develop great hand to eye coordination. Just stand at one end of the room with your child at the other and practicing throwing a ball back and forth. There is nothing complex about this.

DRAWING AND CUTTING

Have your child draw his or her favorite picture. They can use crayons, pencils, or markers. Just allow them to be as creative as possible.

Now, have your child cut the edges of the picture out to hang on the refrigerator. Help them to make cuts if needed. Just remember that the cuts do not have to be perfect. It takes a lot of skill and concentration to cut with scissors while patching.

RED LIGHT, GREEN LIGHT

Color two large cards. Color one card red and the other card green. Have your child stand at one end of the room while you are at the other end of the room. Next, hold up a card in the air for your child to see.

When the card is green, then beckon for your child to come. When you hold up the red card, then your child should immediately stop. Alternate between the two cards and see how quickly your child can react when the cards change.

A more advanced tactic would be for you to write the words "RED" and "GREEN" on the large cards. Your child will need to have the ability to read if you use words instead. Or you can also use flashlights that can reflect red or green lights as an alternative.

ACTIVITY AND COLORING BOOKS

Activity books and coloring books provide some of the easiest nearsighted activities available. If you search through an activity book, there is at least one type of activity that your child likes, whether it is dot to dot puzzles or word search.

You can find these at inexpensive stores and can provide easy activities for your child to do. Depending on the level of severity of your amblyopia, it can take some time for your child to successfully complete a full word search puzzle. However, it can still serve as a great nearsighted activity.

JIGSAW PUZZLES

One of the first activities that we did with my daughter was putting together jigsaw puzzles. However, we found greater success with puzzles that were no more than 10-25 pieces.

If you go for puzzles with 50 or 100 pieces, then this will probably be very frustrating because it was extremely hard for my daughter to be able to distinguish which pieces belong where on the puzzle when they are too small.

If you stick to puzzles with a small number of pieces that are large in size, then it will enable you to have a greater level of success with puzzles. To make it more beneficial for your child, then you may want to consider finding puzzles geared toward a specific character that your child may like. For example, Spiderman® or Barbie® themed puzzles may work well depending on if your child is a boy or girl.

BUBBLE TIME

One of the activities that our pediatric optometrist recommended involved poking bubbles. I am sure that you are familiar with the bubble solution that comes in a bottle that you can purchase from any discount store. It comes with a bubble wand that you can use to blow bubbles through.

As you blow bubbles, have your child use his or her finger to poke as many bubbles as possible. Please note that it is important that they use a finger to poke the bubbles as opposed to the entire hand. This is such an easy to do activity that even a small toddler can do it.

SCRAPBOOKING

Maybe you are already an avid scrap booker. Well, if you can share this hobby with your child, then that can also be something that your child can enjoy as an activity during patching.

Scrapbooking involves doing so many nearsighted activities, like cutting, drawing, coloring, applying stamps or stickers, etc. If you spend your patching time doing scrapbook activities, then there is no doubt that it will offer some benefit.

You can begin by starting a new scrapbooking project of maybe something that your child may have an interest in. Even if you have never done any scrapbooking before, then this is something that you both can easily do together.

VIDEO GAMES

I have not used video games as a patching activity. However, I have heard many parents rave how useful they have been. Primarily, if you already have a personal game system, like a Gameboy®, Nintendo DS®, or even a Leapster®, then you can try them out for their effectiveness.

This method is really designed for older children who like to play games. Since they will most likely play a game anyway, then this can be done during their patching time.

Please note that this method is for small personal game systems more than console style type games (i.e. Playstation® or Xbox® systems) because personal gaming systems utilize hand to eye coordination.

WOOD BLOCKS

This activity works especially well for younger children or toddlers. You may already have a stack of wooden blocks at home that you can use. Have your child stack the set of wood blocks on top of each other until they fall down. Repeat the whole process again.

If your wood blocks contain alphabet letters on them, then you can also have your child make words out of them. This would only work for children who can read.

SLAP JACK

With this exercise, you will only need a deck of playing cards. Deal out the set of cards between all of the players. Have each player pull out a card and place it into a pile. Each player should take a turn.

When a player pulls out the Jack onto the pile of cards, then all players should try to be the first player who "slaps" or hits that card. If you are first to slap the card, then you get the entire pile of cards.

Repeat this until all of the Jacks have been found. The player with the most cards wins the game.

DOMINOES

For small children, stacking dominoes can be a fairly simple activity. However, playing the game of dominoes can be a game that older kids can have fun with as well.

If you feel that the classic game of dominoes may be too advanced for your child, then you may want to try using dominoes that have pictures of characters on them. We were able to get a domino set based on one my daughter's favorite characters, Dora the Explorer.

As an option to playing the game of dominoes, you can have your child stand up the dominoes in a single line. Once completed, have them tap a domino at either end so that they all begin to fall over.

BUILDING WITH LEGOS

You may already own a set of Legos®. Legos® can be a great activity because they allow a child to use their manipulative skills to build anything that they want.

If your child already enjoys playing with Legos®, then you should not have a problem introducing them during patching time. Just allow your child to play as he or she normally does with them during this time.

CLASSIC BOARD GAMES

You can pull out your classic board games, like Checkers®, Monopoly®, or Life®, as they are really great games that work well as near-sighted exercises. Just play them as you normally would when not patching.

However, it may be important for you to go through them very slowly if your child has trouble playing due to their vision. Always make sure that you change up the rules of the game as needed to assist your child if need be.

TRACING LETTERS AND SHAPES

If your child likes to draw, then they may find tracing letters and shapes as a fun activity. If you can find pre-made stencils, then you can have your child stencil letters and shapes. All you will need to do is just to look around for a good stenciling set.

HOUSEHOLD CHORES

This activity will only work for kids who like performing light housework. This is something that I would ask my daughter to do from time to time and was not something that she did on a regular basis.

However, if she was patching and I really needed to do some light household work, then I would have her wash a couple of dishes or make up the bed. Because they both require good hand and eye coordination, then that worked out well as an exercise and also a way for me to get some cleaning done at the same time.

BEAN BAG TOSS

This is just like the classic bean bag toss that you did in grade school as a child. Just find a bean bag. If you don't have one, then you can use a simple Nerf® ball.

Find a couple of small baskets or buckets and put them on the floor. Have your child stand about a foot or so from the baskets and have him or her throw the bean bags into the baskets. As they progress more and more, then move your child farther away from the baskets to practice throwing the bean bags.

BALL AND PADDLE

If you have been to one of the dollar closeout stores, then I am sure that you have seen these paddles that have a string connected to them. On the other end of that string is a ball that is attached. If you already have one of these, then this can serve as a really good activity.

Just have your child practice hitting the ball as much as possible with the paddle. This exercise can be completed by almost any child on their own.

Another alternative to this is to play ping pong. The only issue is whether or not you have access to a ping pong table. Additionally, this may be an even greater challenge if your child is not good at hitting balls with the paddle.

WHO MOVED MY BEANS

This is an easy activity for any child. All you need are two small jars. The ideal size would be baby food jars. Fill one jar with beans or rice. Next, have your child pour the rice and beans into the other jar. Simply go back and forth between the jars pouring the rice or beans.

As an alternative to this technique, you can have your child pick up the beans with their fingers and place it in the jar. Of course, this requires that they be able to see them and are comfortable handling these items. If you child needs a large object to handle, then you can also use coins.

BLURT OUT

To perform this activity, the only thing that you will need is a soccer ball or kickball. Write various letters all over the ball. However, they should be spaced apart. Next, attach a string to the ball so that you can hang it or attach it to the ceiling. Try to make the length of the string long enough so that the ball hangs between your child's chin and waist.

To get started, have your child push the ball back and forth to you. When they receive the ball, then they should read and blurt out all the letters that they see on the ball. They should immediately throw it back to you for you to do the same.

HOMEWORK

If you have a school-aged child, then you will probably at times need to overlap homework time with patch time. Most of the time, your child will have a near-sighted activity as their homework, like reading or writing. So, if your child's vision is advanced enough where they can read and write with their patch on, then you can perform some of your child's homework with the patch on.

However, if your child has problems completing homework with the patch, then this may not work for you. You may limit it to only times when your child has certain activities to complete, like coloring or cutting out objects.

PICK UP STICKS

If you are not familiar with pick up sticks, then let me describe it here. Basically, you will have a bunch of sticks (anywhere ranging from 20 or more sticks). You drop them on a table or desk.

Then, you will take turns with your child to see who can pick up the most sticks. However, the objective of the game is that you cannot move a stick while you are picking up another stick. If you do, you will lose your turn. The person with the most sticks will win the game. I found this game at a discount store for just a couple of dollars.

MAGNETIC DARTS

I was able to find this pretty inexpensive set of magnetic darts that my daughter really enjoys. It has a simple magnetic bulls eye. The only thing that we did is just hang it on a wall.

I would then ask my daughter to target the bulls eye. At first, you can begin only a couple feet a way from the target and then have your child begin to move farther away as their vision steadily increases. Just remember to stay with magnetic darts.

If you use real darts, then this can pose a huge danger to both you and your child.

GO FISH

I guess most of us grew up on the card game of "Go Fish". To use this as a near sighted activity, then we really do not have to do much. Just deal of the set of cards. You can go with each player having 5 or 7 cards to begin with. Ask your child if they if a certain kind of card. If they do, then take the card from them.

If they don't have the card, then you would need to "Go Fish" or draw a new card from the stack. Do this until all cards are gone.

LITE BRITE

If you have an old Lite Brite® game, then you can also use this during patching time. I have a travel Lite Brite system that comes complete with all the different pegs. I bought this at the local Walmart® in my area. The system comes with several pegs of different colors.

Just have your child, practice inserting all the pegs in the holes. Let them be creative and come up with their own design. When all is done, turn the light on to view the design.

IT'S MUSIC TIME

You can add even more fun to your patch time with the use of music. Just gather all the musical instruments that you have. Toy pianos, xylophones, recorders, flutes, and drums are perfect items for this activity.

Make up your own songs to sing and dance to. This will be so much fun and your child will be able to relieve any anxiety and frustration that they have during the patching session.

My daughter also enjoys practicing the piano with her patch. We have a full size piano at home that we just allow her to practice on any way that she sees fit.

WATER TIME

If you have children who love taking baths and playing in water, then you can also perform some water activities while patching. Just fill the tub with water and add bath toys (like ducks, frogs, etc) that your child can play with during this time.

Just be cautious if you have a small child or toddler when playing with water while patching. You want the activity to be fun; however, you don't want to pose a danger to them in the process. If your child has a problem seeing well when patching, then this activity may not be for you.

I SPY

I am not sure if you have heard of the "I Spy" games. However, we have used both the "I Spy" card game as well as used a variation of it that does not require anything.

For this, have your child focus on an item that is in the same room. Next, have your child describe the item. They would say, "I Spy something green" as an example. Then have them continue describing the item until you figure out what it is. If you have "I Spy" cards, then you can ask them to pick out an item in the cards to describe as an alternative.

EYE AND HAND COORDINATION

With this activity, you will only need a set of matching cards to complete it. You can use memory cards or a deck of playing cards. To begin, choose 5 set of mates. Create two rows of cards. Put one mate on each row. Then, give your child a pencil. Have your child start with the first card in the first row. Touch the center of the card with the pencil.

Then, have your child find the mate on the second row and touch the center of that. Complete this for all cards. As you get more advanced, use as many mates as possible to complete the exercise and see how quickly your child can do it. Also, be sure your child does this exercise using both the left and right hand.

WHICH FINGER?

This is a simple exercise that does not require any form of equipment. To complete this exercise, raise your hands so that they are facing your child's face. Your hands should only be a foot apart from each other. Tell your child that the first finger is "number 1" and so on until you count all 10 fingers.

Now, tell your child that you will call out the finger number and your child should immediately focus their eyes on that finger. You will need to alternate what is called between your fingers and hands. Make sure that your child moves their eyes and not their hand toward the finger that is being called.

BALL AND LEVER

To complete this exercise, all you need is a small ball. A tennis ball should be fine. You will just need an item like a lever or something that can technically launch a ball in the air. The objective of this exercise will be to launch a ball in the air for your child to catch.

However, the difference here is that you will tell your child to catch it with either the left or right hand each time the ball is thrown while it is in mid-air.

BALANCING ACT

This is an activity that would work better for older kids as opposed to young toddlers .To get started, all you need to have available is a balance board or a balance beam. You will just need to hang a softball or tennis ball from the ceiling. Be sure to suspend it so that it hangs at your child's eye level. It should begin to slightly rotate.

Next, have your child stand on a balance board and try to hold their balance as they fixate their eyes on the ball. This activity may be a challenge if your child has trouble walking or cannot maintain their balance.

PATTERNS

This is an easy exercise that can also be a bit challenging as well. To begin, you will either need a set of wooden shapes or else you can make the shapes yourself. The shapes will need to be a set of circles, squares, and triangles.

Sit at a table or on the floor with your child and create a pattern with the shapes. For example, you can have a pattern of 2 circles, 1 square, and then 1 triangle. Let your child observe the pattern for a few seconds. Now, use a box to cover up the pattern.

Ask your child to recreate the pattern for you with their set of shapes. For a more advanced method, rotate or connect the shapes and have your child reproduce these from memory.

SHAPE CUT OUTS

Prior to completing this activity, you need to cut out various shapes (squares, circles, etc) from construction paper. Once you have your shapes ready, cut a piece of that shape out. Do this for a minimum of 5 shapes.

Then, lay out your shapes and the pieces that were cut out and ask your child to identify which piece belongs to which shape. This is almost a form of using shapes as puzzle pieces.

WHICH IS NOT LIKE THE OTHER

If you can find activity books or children's magazines that include these types of games, then this would be great. However, if you cannot, then you may find printable sheets for these on the Internet.

Basically, what you want to do is to find two pictures that look exactly alike, however, they contain slight differences between the two that may not be so easy to notice. An example would be if you had two pictures that were alike, but one of the pictures has a bird and the other doesn't.

Ask your child to locate the differences between the two pictures. Be sure to give hints if needed to find the differences.

HIDDEN ITEMS

For this activity, it may be difficult to find a picture that would be suitable. However, the objective of this is to locate an item in a picture that is not easily noticed.

Then ask your child to find that hidden item. This exercise works very well with "I Spy"® playing cards. "I Spy"® playing cards have present several objects presented on one card that you can choose from. These can easily be purchased at any discount store.

PARTIAL ITEMS

I love this activity because it makes your child's brain work even faster. The goal of this activity is to have your child identify an object or word when only part of it is presented to them. The hardest part will be for you to either locate cards that you can use or to make the cards yourself.

I made some using the Windows Paint tool on my computer. However, here are examples of words that illustrate the concept of partial words. You would need to just ask your child to read off words like these for you. If you notice, some parts of the word are grayed out. Of course, pictures can be used as opposed to words for children who cannot read.

egg

heart

JUMP ALL BUT ONE GAMES

This is a game that my daughter really enjoys to play. It is a game that we purchased at one of the old country stores. It includes a wooden triangle that contains 15 holes. There are also 14 - 15 tees like the kind that you play with golf that come with game.

You first start off placing 14 tees into the holes. The goal is for you to jump over the tees like you do in the game of Checkers®. Each time you jump over one, remove it from off the wooden board.

You will want to get to the point when you cannot jump over any more. The ultimate goal is to only have one remain, but that is more difficult than you think. Have your child try this game a couple of times on their own.

I hope that you enjoyed the information presented in this book. This book was strictly written with you in mind in an effort to provide information for those who wear eye patches due to a lazy eye condition. I hope through this book that you have gained more knowledge that can assist you obtaining improved vision through eye patching.

It is my intent that you would be able to use some of the activities presented in this book with your child during patching. Hopefully, these activities can spark new ideas for other activities that you can try out with your child in the process.

Although eye patching can be very labor intensive, science has proven that it can be very effective in the fight against lazy eye or amblyopia. Since we all have to do it given our various condition, then let's make the best use of this time as much as possible.

It does not have to be a horrible experience that your child remembers their entire lifetime. It can be an experience that they cherish when they think of the wonderful quality time that you spent with them playing games and having fun.

ACTIVITY CHART

Fill out the exercises that are done per day and indicate the days that they are performed within a specified week.

Week: _____

Activity	Sun	Mon	Tues	Wed	Thurs	Fri	Sat

Areas of Difficulty:

_____

_____

Observations:

_____

_____